Keto Seafood Cookbook

Delicious keto-style seafood recipes

Sommario

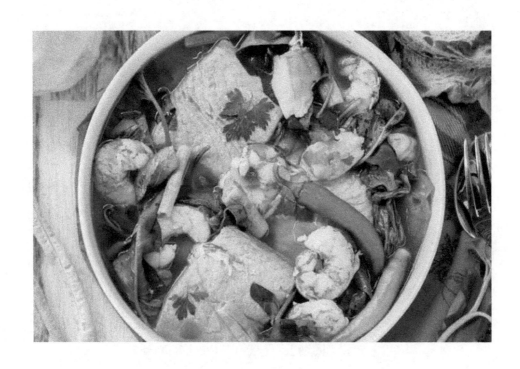

INTRODUCTION

Welcome to this fantastic journey into the delights of the sea.

The sea has always been a source of sustenance for all peoples since ancient times, and in this book I wanted to enclose the quick and easy recipes to prepare the products of the sea in keto style, great for a vitamin intake but also protein, ideal for keeping healthy, but also with a fitness body.

The recipes are designed for everyone, beginners and not, you will find fish, seafood made in many ways.

But let's not get lost in so many words and start preparing these delicious dishes right away.

SEAFOOD RECIPES

WHITEFISH WITH PARMESAN AND PESTO

Ingredients

- 2 white fish fillets, about 6 oz each

- 3 Tbsp pine nuts

- 2 Tbsp parmesan

- ¼ tsp finely chopped garlic (1 garlic clove)

- 1 tsp basil pesto

- 1 ½ Tbsp mayonnaise

Instructions

1   Preheat the oven or toaster at 400°F / 200C. Spray individual pans with nonstick spray or olive oil (use a large saucepan if you do not have 1).

2   Remove fish from the refrigerator and let them reach the temperature while the oven is overheating. (It is essential to have the fish at room temperature. Otherwise, it will not be cooked until the lid is too brown).

3   Use a large chef's knife to finely chop the pine nuts and chop the garlic. Mix chopped pine nuts, parmesan cheese, chopped garlic, basil pesto, and mayonnaise.

4   Use a rubber scraper to spread the crust mixture evenly over the surface of each fish fillet. Apply it to the crust mixture.

5   Cooked fish for 10 to 15 min, until the fish is firm and the crust mixture begins to brown a little. (I cooked the fish pieces on the picture for 13 min). Serve hot.

Servings: 2; **Prep time:**30 min

WIRE CREAM AIL

Ingredients

- 1 Tbsp olive oil

- 1 lb (500 g) shrimp, with or without tail

- Salt and pepper to taste

- 2 Tbsp unsalted butter

- 6 garlic cloves, finely chopped

- ½ cup dry white wine or chicken broth

- 1 ½ cups of skimmed cream

- ½ cup grated fresh parmesan cheese

- 2 Tbsp chopped fresh parsley

Instructions

1   Heat the oil in a large skillet over medium heat. Season shrimp with salt and pepper and fry for 1-2 min per side until well cooked and pink. Transfer to a bowl; put aside.

2   Melt the butter in the same pan. Fry the garlic until fragrant (about 30 seconds). For the white wine or broth; reduce by half while scraping the lower parts of the pan.

3   Reduce heat to medium, add cream and simmer, stirring occasionally. Season with salt and pepper.

4   Add parmesan sauce and simmer for a minute until cheese melts and sauce thickens.

5   Add the shrimp in the pan, sprinkle with parsley.

Prep time: 10 min;

Macros: Cal 488 | Carbs 4 g | Protein 30 g | Fat 44 g Saturated Fat 25 g | Cholesterol 234 mg | Sodium 110 mg Potassium 223 mg | Vitamin A: 1765 IU | Vitamin C: 9.2 mg | Calcium: 375 mg | Iron: 2.8 mg

FILLET WITH GARLIC AND SHRIMP

Ingredients

- 2 lean beef fillets or steak of your choice

- salt and pepper

- Tbsp olive oil

- 1 Tbsp butter

- 1 lb of shrimp, shelled and evaded

- 3 cloves of garlic, finely chopped

Garlic butter:

- ¼ cup soft butter

- 3 cloves of garlic, finely chopped

- 1 tsp chopped thyme

- 1 tsp minced rosemary

- 1 tsp minced oregano

Instructions

1   Place a medium skillet over high heat. Add olive oil and butter. Add the steaks. Cook on each side for 3 min or until golden brown.

2   Lower the temperature to medium to low. Cook the steaks. Remove and place on a plate.

3   Reduce the fire to a low. Add shrimp and garlic and cook for 2 to 3 minutes until they become opaque. Add the steaks back to the pan. Mix the butter, garlic, and chopped fresh herbs.

Prep time:5 min; **Servings:** 6

Macros: Cal 699 Lipids 32g49% Saturated fat 10 g 5g Carbs 1 g oFiber 1 g of sugar 94 g of protein

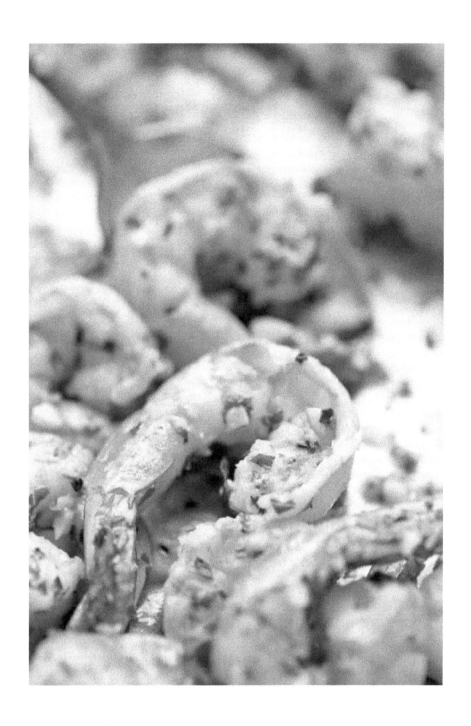

KETO TUNA MORNAY

Ingredients

- 1 batch of keto cheese sauce

- 400 g broccoli florets (14 oz)

- 425 g tuna, drained (15 oz)

- 100 g grated cheddar (4 oz)

Instructions

1 Preheat the oven to 180° C / 350° F.

2 Boil the broccoli until they are soft; do not boil them too much, as they will cook a bit more in the oven.

3 Place the broccoli in a baking dish evenly over the tuna. Pour the prepared cheese sauce and sprinkle with grated cheese.

4 Bake for 15-20 min until golden and bubbling. Let cool 5 min before serving.

Prep time: 15 min; **Servings:** 4

Macros: Cal 632 | Carbs 9 g | Protein 34g | Fat 51 g | Fiber 2g | Sugar 1 g | Net Carbs 7 g

SHRIMP PAPER

Ingredients

- 2 lbs of shrimp, 907 g

- 16 cherry tomatoes, cut in half

- 2 small zucchini

- 1 yellow pepper, cut into pieces

- 2 Tbsp olive oil

- 2 crushed garlic cloves

- 1 tsp salt

- 1 tsp pepper

- 4 slices of lemon

- 1 Tbsp finely chopped parsley

Instructions

How to cook the pack of shrimp sheets on a grill

1   Prepare the shrimp and vegetables as follows and wrap the aluminum containers.

2   Bake shrimp paper packets for about 10 to 15 min on a hot grill or until vegetables are cooked through. Serve hot and sprinkle with parsley chopped and lemon juice.

Cooking with oven shrimp packages

1   Preheat oven to 400°F

2   Cut 4 large foil sheets, about 12-15 inches long.

3   Mix shrimp, tomatoes, and zucchini in olive oil, garlic, salt, and pepper and let stand in for 15 min and stir again.

4   Divide the shrimp and vegetable mixture over the pieces of aluminum and cover with a slice of lemon.

5   Fold aluminum wrappers over shrimps and vegetables to cover the food completely, then fold up and down to close.

6   Bake 15 to 20 min or until vegetables and shrimp are cooked through.

7   Serve hot and sprinkle with parsley chopped and lemon juice.

Prep time:10 min; **Servings:** 4

Macros: Cal 326 10 g oFat Saturated fat 1 g 8g Carbs 1 g oFiber 3 g of sugar 48 g of protein

ATLANTIC COD WITH HERB BUTTER AND HERBS

Ingredients

- 6 Tbsp unsalted butter, sweet

- 1/ 2 tsp garlic, finely chopped

- 1 tsp fresh parsley, finely chopped

- 1 tsp fresh thyme leaves

- tsp fresh basil, finely chopped

- ¼ tsp sea salt

- Tbsp extra virgin olive oil

- 6 Atlantic cod fillets of 4 oz

- Sea salt and black pepper to taste

- Fresh parsley, chopped, to decorate

Instructions

4   Prepare garlic and herb butter by all ingredients in a medium bowl. Stir until garlic, herbs, and salt are evenly distributed over the soft butter.

5   Transfer the butter mixture to the center of a plastic sheet and form a stem. Wrap them up in the refrigerator for 15 to 20 minutes to make them firm.

6   Heat the olive oil in a skillet over medium heat. Dry the cod fillets with paper towels and season with salt and black pepper.

7   Add the steaks to skillet and cook for 2 to 3 min or until golden brown. Cover each steak with an equal amount of herb butter and another 3-4 min While cooking, place the butter on the fillets as it melts.

8   Remove from heat and transfer to individual dishes for serving. Sprinkle with melted herb butter and garnish with fresh chopped parsley, if desired.

Prep time:5 min; **Servings:** 6

Macros: Total Carbs 0.43 g Fiber 0.1 g Net Carbs 0.33 g Protein 43%

Fat content: 56% Carbs 1%

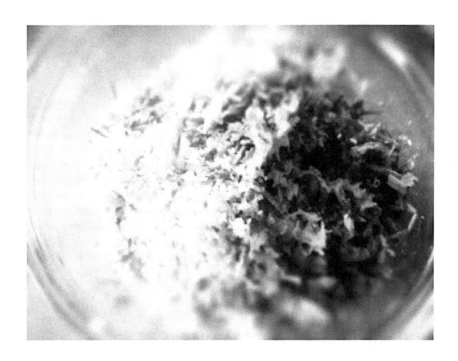

HEALTHY OKRA SEAFOOD

Ingredients

- ½ cup cassava flour

- ⅓ cup speech juice

- ½ cup chopped celery

- 1 cup chopped onion

- 1 cup green pepper, seeded and minced

- 1 clove garlic, minced

- ½ lb sliced chicken and apple sausage

- 4 cups beef broth

- 2 cups of water

- 1 Tbsp coconut amino acids

- 1 ½ - 2 tsp salt

- 1 Tbsp Louisiana hot sauce

- 1 tsp Cajun spice blend

- 2 bay leaves

- ¼ tsp dried thyme leaves

- 1 can (14.5 g) diced tomatoes in juice

- 2 tsp divided gumbo-lime powder, optional

- 1 Tbsp avocado oil or more fat bacon

- 1 pack of 10 g oFrozen frost frozen okra

- 1 Tbsp white vinegar

- 8 g of drained crabmeat

- 1 ½ lbs medium uncooked shrimp, shelled and thawed

- Fresh parsley, minced, optional

Instructions

1   Heat ⅓ cup bacon in a large Dutch oven over medium heat. Sprinkle with cassava, and a smooth dough appears. Cook this mixture, stirring almost constantly, for about 30 min, or until it

turns to deep amber color. Do not let it burn; make this process happen slowly and gradually.

2   Add celery, onion, pepper, and garlic to a food processor and press several times until the mixture is finely chopped.

3   When the roux has a vibrant amber color, add the mixture of celery, onion, pepper, and garlic; Add the sliced sausage. Mix well, then add 1 cup water and beat well. Bring the mixture to a boil over medium heat and cook for about 15 min. If necessary, add the second cup of water to prevent the dough from sticking to the bottom of the Dutch oven.

4   Meanwhile, boil 4 cups of beef broth in a medium-sized saucepan. Add the coconut amino acids, salt, hot sauce, Cajun spices, bay leaves, dried thyme, and diced tomatoes. Simmer for 2 hours over medium heat. If you have a gumbo girl add 1 tsp to the soup after 1 hour.

5   Meanwhile, heat 1 Tbsp avocado oil in the saucepan used to heat the beef broth. Add the thawed okra and vinegar and cook on medium heat for 15 min or until they are sticky and soft. Stir the okra with crabmeat and shrimp. Simmer for 45 minutes over low

heat. If you have a fillet of okra, add the remaining tsp just before serving.

Servings: 6; **Prep time:**45 min

Macros: Cal 273 Lipids 13g20% Saturated fat 4 g Carbs 12g4% 2g8% oFiber 3g3% sugar 24 g48% protein

FRIED SALMON WITH CREAMY SAUCE

Ingredients

4. 6 pieces of salmon (about 4 g each)

5. 1 Tbsp chopped fresh dill

6. Olive oil

7. Salt and pepper to taste

For the sauce:

8. 1 Tbsp chopped fresh dill

9. ⅓ cup sour cream

10. 2 Tbsp mayonnaise

11. 1 tsp Dijon mustard

12. 1 Tbsp chopped capers

13. ½ lemon juice and zest

14. Salt and pepper to taste

Instructions

1   Make the sauce by mixing all the ingredients in a bowl; leave at room temperature while you prepare the salmon.

2   Preheat the oven to 400°F.

3   Place the salmon on a baking sheet lined with foil. Brush each piece with olive oil. Sprinkle with salt, pepper, and dill.

4   Bake 10 min.

5   Increase the temperature to 450°F and cook another 5-8 min.

6   Serve with a spoonful of sauce and garnish with dill and capers.

Prep time:5 min; **Servings:** 6

Macros: Cal 348 Lipids 27g Saturated fat 2g Carbs 1g 27 g protein

KETO CAJUN TRINITY

Ingredients

- 2 tsp

- 1 full celery, finely chopped

- ½ cup chopped mixed pepper

- 1 shallot

- 2 garlic cloves, finely chopped

- sea salt and black pepper, to taste

- 1 large egg

- 2 Tbsp mayonnaise

- 1 Tbsp Worcestershire sauce

- 1 tsp spicy brown mustard

- 1 tsp hot sauce

- ½ cup grated Parmesan cheese

- ½ cup crushed pork rind

- 1 lb of crab meat in pieces, without shell

- 2 Tbsp olive oil

Instructions

1. Heat to the frying pan over medium heat. Heat the butter in the pan and add celery, pepper, shallots, garlic, sea salt, and black pepper. Bake until vegetables is transparent and soft, about 10 min

2. Mix the egg, mayonnaise, Worcestershire, spicy brown mustard, and spicy sauce in a large bowl. Add the baked vegetables, and all ingredients are well absorbed. Mix the Parmesan and the pork rind. Fold the crab into the mixture.

3. Cover a large baking sheet with parchment paper. Form the crab mixture into 8 patties. Place the patties on the prepared baking sheet and refrigerate for 1 to 2 hours.

4. Cooked in olive oil in a large skillet over medium heat until crab cakes on both sides are golden and crisp.

Prep time: 15 min; **Servings:** 2

Macros: Cal 412 Fat 28 g Carbs 4 g Fiber 1 g

CREAMY KETO SHRIMP WITH MEDITERRANEAN ZOODLES

Ingredients

- 2 zucchini medium size, spiralized

- 1 lb of shrimp, uncooked, deveined and without tail

- 1.5 Tbsp tomato puree

- 4 oz cream cheese

- ½ cup half and half

- 2 Tbsp thyme

- 2 Tbsp garlic powder

- 2 oregano Tbsp

- 1 Tbsp parsley flakes

- 1 Tbsp onion powder

- 1 tsp turmeric

- 1 Tbsp red pepper flakes

- ½ cup grated Parmesan cheese

Instructions

1. Preheat the oven to 400° F. Melt butter in a cast iron skillet and add zoodles and shrimp.

2. Mix the herbs, cream cheese, butter, and half and half in a small saucepan over medium heat. Stir regularly.

3. Cook the noodles and shrimp for 5-8 min Remove the sauce and add it to shrimp and zoodles. Stir, add Parmesan cheese, and cook another 10 min.

Prep time:10 min; **Servings:** 4

Macros: Cal 381 | Carbs 8 g | Protein 31.8 g | Fat 21.9 g | Saturated Fat 12.8 g | Sodium 434 mg Fiber 4.2 g

GARLIC SQUID

Ingredients

- 10oz / 300g Squid

- ½ lemon juice

- 2 Tbsp olive oil

- 2 cloves garlic

- ⅓ cup boneless olives

- ½ cup arugula

- 2 Tbsp tomato puree

- 1 Tbsp dried basil

- ground pepper

- Parmesan cheese

Instructions

1   Cook the squid in a saucepan with a little water for 3-4 min, covered with a lid. Make sure the squid is ready. Remove the extra water and add the lemon juice and olive oil.

2   Add the tomato puree and add 2 Tbsp water if necessary. Squeeze the garlic, add the dried basil and cracked pepper.

3   Garnish with parmesan or add another type of cheese.

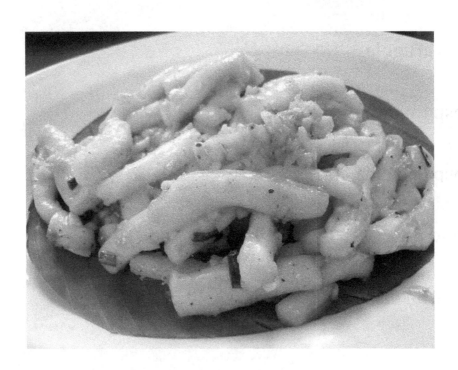

KETO SHRIMP FAJITAS

Ingredients

- 1.5 lbs Fresh shrimp

- 1 large yellow pepper, finely sliced

- 1 medium green pepper, sliced thinly

- small red peppers sliced thinly

- 1 little chili, cut into thin slices

- medium red onions sliced thinly

- jalapenos in thin slices

- 3/4 cup finely chopped celery stalks

Adobo (divided):

- 3 Lime gold lime, juice extract

- ¼ tsp garlic powder

- ½ tsp chili powder

- ½ tsp Spanish pepper

- ¼ tsp ground cumin

- ⅓ cup olive oil

- Salt and black pepper ground to taste

Instructions

1   Wash the shrimp thoroughly with water. Remove the bowl, head, and vein. Keep the tails intact. Dry with paper towels. Put aside.

2   In a bowl, mix olive oil, gold lime juice, garlic powder, chili powder, Spanish pepper, cumin, salt, and black pepper.

3   Pour marinade over the pepper and shrimp slices. Marinate for at least 15 min

4   Spread pepper, jalapeño pepper, celery, and half of the red onions in a baking dish and sprinkle with marinade. Bake at 400° F for 5 min.

5   Add the shrimp to the dish. Bake for 5 to 8 min..

6   Heat tortillas.

7   Serve with avocado slices and sour cream on the side.

Prep time:20 min; **Servings:** 8

Macros: Cal 158 | Carbs 5 g | Protein 13 g | Fat 10 g Saturated Fat 1 g | Polyunsaturated Fat 1 g | Monounsaturated Fat 7 g | Cholesterol 101 mg | Sodium 85 mg Potassium 290 mg | Fiber 3g | Sugar 1 g | Vitamin A: 650 IU | Vitamin C: 82.5 mg | Calcium: 50 mg | Iron: 0.9 mg

SHRIMP ALLA VODKA

Ingredients

- 1 lb of raw shrimp, shelled and sliced

- 4 g oFinely sliced prosciutto, diced

- Box of 28 g of organic crushed tomatoes (no added salt / low-carb)

- 15 oz organic diced tomatoes (no added salt / low Carbs)

- 1 cup thick whipped cream

- ⅓ cup vodka (without taste)

- 5 fresh basil leaves

- 2 garlic cloves, finely chopped

- 1 Tbsp olive oil

- A pinch of salt and pepper

- Parmesan grated to cover

- zucchini, spiral "spaghetti" about ½ per person

Instructions

1. Heat a large skillet over medium heat, add olive oil and ham. Fry the bacon for 2 min and add garlic to cook for another minute. Be careful not to brown the garlic. Remove from heat and scrape all browned parts of the bottom of the pan.

2. Slowly reduce vodka, then add tomato sauce, dried basil, parsley, heavy cream, salt, and pepper. Cook over medium heat with lid overstuffed for 25 min, stirring occasionally.

3. While the sauce is boiling, you can prepare your zucchini noodles or "zoodles." Cut each end of the zucchini and spiralize. Cut into traditional spaghetti pieces and set aside.

4. After boiling for 25 min, add the sauce and cook another 5 min

5. Add zucchini noodles to your plate, top with shrimp and grated parmesan cheese. Garnish with fresh basil leaves.

Prep time: 5 min; **Servings:** 2

Macros: Cal212 Lipids 11g17% Saturated fat 8g50% Carbs 7g2% 2g8% oFiber 3g3% sugar 12 g of 24% protein

CRAB OMELET WITH AVOCADO AND HERBS

Ingredients

- 3 eggs

- 1 tsp chopped parsley

- 1 tsp chopped chives

- ½ tsp sea salt or kosher

- ½ tsp ground black pepper

- 1 Tbsp butter

- ½ oz grated Parmesan about 2 Tbsp

- 2 oz crab meat into about ½ cup pieces

- 1 green onion, finely sliced

- ½ sliced avocado

- 1 Tbsp sour cream

Instructions

1. Break the eggs in a small bowl. Add the onions, parsley, salt, and pepper

2. Place a 10-inch nonstick skillet over medium heat, add the butter, and stir until it melts.

3. Pour the beaten eggs in the pan. Shake the pan to cover the bottom of the pan. Fry the eggs over medium heat until the edges are firm, and the medium is barely cooked for 3-4 min Deflate the big bubbles with the teeth of a fork.

4. Sprinkle half of the Parmesan on half of the tortilla. Cover the crabmeat with cheese and green onions. Place the avocado on the green onions and cover with remaining Parmesan cheese.

5. Using a spatula, fold the empty half of the eggs to form a semicircle. Remove from heat and transfer to a plate. Sprinkle with fresh herbs to taste and decorate with a Tbsp sour cream. Serve immediately.

Prep time: 10 min; **Servings:** 1

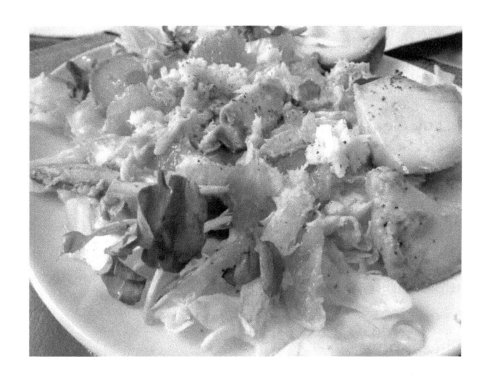

SALMON BROCCOLI FUN BAG

Ingredients

- ½ cup broccoli, minced

- 1 celery stalk, finely chopped

- ¼ leek, cut, clean and cut

- A pinch of chopped fresh rosemary, chili powder, and curry powder

- Cayenne pepper to taste (optional)

- g of wild salmon

- ¼ sliced avocado

- Coriander, sliced green onions and sliced watermelon radish to taste

- 1-2 Tbsp cerebral octane oil

- Cooked and cooled white rice (optional), flavored with ground turmeric

Instructions

5   Cook the salmon using your preferred method (poaching is recommended).

6   While the salmon cooks, prepare the base of the leek with broccoli. Generously season a pot of water with salt and boil. Add broccoli, celery, and leek and cook 10 min or until tender.

7   Drain the vegetables and save about ½ cup the cooking liquid.

8   Transfer the vegetables to a blender and mix until puree, add a Tbsp boiling water at a time until it reaches a consistency of the vegetable puree. (You can also do it in your pot with a hand blender). Add rosemary, chili powder, curry powder, and cayenne pepper (if used) and mix well.

9   Put the broccoli leek base in a bowl and cover with rice, cooked salmon, avocado, and remaining vegetables. Spray with cerebral octane oil and serve hot.

Prep time:20 min**; Servings:** 1

Macros: Cal 374 Fat 20.4 g Carbs 14 g Fiber 6.3 g Protein 26.6 g Carbs 7.7 g

SALMON WITH TOMATO AND CUCUMBER

Ingredients

- 5 oz wild salmon fillets, skinless

- 1 ball oFennel, thickly sliced

- 1 large cucumber

- ½ cup boneless green olives

- 3 Tbsp butter or herb butter

- Fresh thyme leaves

- 2 extra virgin olive oil Tbsp

Instructions

1. Preheat the oven to 350° F.

2. Place the salmon on the fennel and the dotted ghee on the salmon. Sprinkle fresh thyme leaves on top.

3. Bake the salmon in the oven for 15 min

4. While the salmon is in the oven, twist the cucumber into noodles and allow the excess water to drain by pressing gently.

5. Put the noodles in a bowl and dress them with extra virgin olive oil.

6. Remove the salmon from the oven.

7. Put the noodles on a plate and put the salmon on it. Add the green olives and sprinkle with salt to taste.

Prep time: 10 min; **Servings:** 2

Macros: Cal 502.4 Protein 38.9 g Carbs 15.6 g Fiber 5.32 g Carbs 8.6 g Sugar 7.1 g Fat 31.6 g Saturated Fat 4.38 g

TANDOORI OVEN SALMON

Ingredients

5. 2 4 oz wild salmon fillets

6. g of unsweetened natural coconut milk yogurt

7. 1 Tbsp raw apple cider vinegar

8. 1 Tbsp avocado oil

9. 1 tsp ground ginger or 1 inch fresh ginger mixed

10. 1 tsp ground turmeric

11. 1 tsp green cardamom seeds

12. 1 tsp Ceylon cinnamon

13. 1 tsp cloves

14. 1 tsp cumin seeds

Instructions

7. Prepare the tandoori salmon. Mix the coconut yogurt in a bowl with all the herbs. Put the salmon in the pan and cover. Leave to marinate for 30 min (either at the counter if you plan to cook immediately, or in the fridge if you plan to cook later).

8. Preheat the oven to 350° F. Cover a baking sheet with aluminum foil.

9. Remove the salmon from the marinade and place the skin on the baking sheet.

10. Bake for 5 min Lift the oven rack and grill the salmon for 2-3 min until a light brown crust appears.

Prep time:15 min; **Servings:** 2

Macros: Cal 432 Protein 34 g Carbs 22.1 g Fiber 8.2 g Sugar 7.8 g Carbs 13.9 g Fat 23 g Saturated Fat 10 g

WILD SALMON OVEN WITH ASPARAGUS AND FENNEL

Ingredients

- 21 oz wild salmon (keta/king/sockeye)

- cups of asparagus

- ½ cup fennel, cut into thin slices

- medium avocados

- 1 Tbsp coconut amino acids

- 1 Tbsp dried seaweed

- 1 tsp Himalayan pink salt

- 1 Tbsp fresh lemon juice

- 1 extra virgin olive oil Tbsp

- Fennel leaves

- Chili flakes (optional)

Instructions

1. Put the salmon in the large bowl, then add the ingredients for the marinade. Amino coconut, dried seaweed, honey, salt, and lemon juice. Mix well and let stand for 20 min

2. Preheat the oven to 350° F.

3. Steamed asparagus and let them cool.

4. Put the sliced fennel in a heat-resistant pan and add the salmon

5. Place the baking sheet in the center of the oven and bake for about 10 min until it is cooked through.

6. Cut them in half and cut the avocados, place them on a plate or serving plate and transfer the salmon to the fennel.

7. Sprinkle with extra virgin olive oil and garnish with fennel leaves, chili flakes, and Himalayan pink salt to taste.

Prep time: 15 min; **Servings:** 4

Macros: Cal 537.7 Protein 50.9 g Carbs 38.1 g Fiber 24.9g Sugar 11.9 g Fat 24.6 g Saturated Fat 1.55 g

KETO CEVICHE

Ingredients

- Fresh halibut from the wild, cubed (preferably sushi grade)

- 1 lime juice

- 2 brain octane oil tsp

- A pinch of Himalayan pink salt

- 1 small avocado, diced

- 1 organic green onion, thinly sliced

- 1 Tbsp chopped fresh organic coriander

- Optional: 2 Tbsp diced pickled radish

Instructions

3. Combine lime juice, brain octane oil, and salt in a medium bowl.

4. Put the rest of the ingredients in the bowl and stir gently.

5. Divide into 2 portions.

Prep time: 15 min **Servings:** 2

Macros: Cal 198 Protein 20 g Carbs 2 g Fiber 2 g Sugar 0 g Fat 10 g
Saturated Fat 5 g

COD IN THE PAN

Ingredients

- 2 ½ lbs of cod fillets

- Tbsp unsalted butter, sliced

- seasoning

- ¼ tsp garlic powder

- ½ tsp table salt

- ¼ tsp ground pepper

- ¾ tsp ground pepper

- A few lemon slices

- Herbs, parsley or coriander

Instructions

1   Combine the herbal ingredients in a small bowl.

2   Cut the cord into small pieces, if desired. Season all sides of the cod with the herbs.

3   Heat 2 Tbsp butter in a large skillet over medium-high heat. As soon as the butter melts, add the cod to the pan. Cook for 2 min

4   Lower the heat to medium. Turn the cod over, cover with the rest of the butter and cook for another 3-4 min

5   The butter melts completely, and the fish boils. (Do not overcook the cod, it will soften and collapse completely).

6   Sprinkle the cod with fresh lemon juice. Cover with fresh herbs if desired. Serve immediately.

Prep time:5 min; **Servings:** 4

Macros: Cal 294 Fat 18 g Saturated fat 11 g Cholesterol 118 mg Sodium 385 mg Potassium 712 mg Protein 30 g

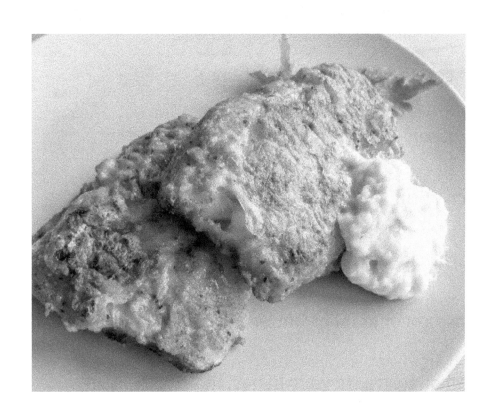

LEMON FISH CAKE WITH AVOCADO SAUCE

Ingredients

- 1 lb of boneless raw fish (preferably local and game)

- ¼ cup coriander (leaves and stems)

- Pinch of salt

- A pinch of chili flakes

- 1-2 garlic cloves (optional)

- 1-2 Tbsp coconut oil or butter fed on frying grass

- Neutral oil to grease your hands, like avocado oil

- 2 ripe avocados

- 1 lemon, juiced

- Pinch of salt

- 2 Tbsp water

Instructions

4. In a food processor, add the fish, herbs, garlic (if used), salt, chili, and fish. Blitz until everything is evenly combined.

5. In a large skillet over medium heat, add the coconut oil or butter and stir to cover.

6. Oil your hands and roll the fish mixture into 6 patties.

7. Add cakes to the hot pan. Cook on both sides until golden and cooked through.

8. While the fish cakes are cooked, add all the ingredients for the dipping sauce (from the lemon juice) in a small food processor or blender and mix until the dough is smooth and creamy. Try the mixture and add more lemon juice or salt if necessary.

9. When the fish cakes are cooked, serve them hot with a dipping sauce.

Servings: 6; **Prep time:** 15 min

Macros: Cal 69 Fat 6.5 g Saturated Fat 1.9 g Cholesterol 6 mg Sodium 54 mg Total Carbs 2.7 g Fiber 2.1g Sugar 0.2 g Carbs 0.6 g Protein 1.1 g

TOMATO BROTH COD POACHED

Ingredients

- 1 lb wild-caught cod fillet, cut into 3-inch squares

- A 28 oz can of organic peeled whole tomatoes (BPA free), drained

- 1.5 cups pastured chicken broth

- pinch of saffron (about 15 threads)

- 2 bay leaves

- 3 avocado oil Tbsp

- Sea salt to taste

Instructions

1. Add the oil to a pan over medium heat. Put the peeled tomatoes in the pan with your hands. Add broth, saffron, bay leaf, and salt to taste.

2. Bring the broth over low heat over medium heat and reduce the heat.

3. Add the cod fillets and cover, simmer for 5-7 min, or only until the fish begins to crumble.

4. Serve the fish with tomato broth.

Servings: 2 **Prep time:** 20 min

Macros: Cal 167 Fat 10.3 g Saturated Fat 1 g Cholesterol 35 mg Sodium 100 mg Total Carbs 1.6 g Dietary Fiber 0.4 g Sugar 0 g Protein 18 g Calcium: 7 mg Potassium 65 mg

KETO FISH AND CHIPS

Ingredients

- 250 g firm white fish, preferably cod

- ⅓ cup sour cream

- tsp apple cider vinegar

- cloves of garlic passed through a press

- Kosher salt to taste

- ½ cup whey protein isolate

- 1 tsp of baking powder

- ¼ tsp garlic powder

- 1 / 4-1 / 2 tsp kosher salt to taste

- 1 egg

- 1 Tbsp sour cream or coconut cream

- 2 tsp apple cider vinegar

- coconut oil or cooking oil of your choice

- 1 batch oFries with 8 jicama tortillas

- 1 bunch of our keto mayonnaise

- lemon

- vinegar

Instructions

7. Mix sour cream (or coconut), vinegar, garlic, and season with salt. Cut the fish through the meat grain into strips about 2.5 cm wide and add them to the cream marinade. Treat and allow to cool for 2 hours, preferably overnight.

8. Prepare your frying station by adding enough oil to a skillet or saucepan to be about ½ inch deep. You can save a lot oFat by using a narrower pan and frying them in batches. Heat the oil over medium / low heat while stirring the fish.

9. Combine whey protein, baking powder, garlic powder, and salt in a shallow dish or dish. Beat the egg in a second dish or a plate with cream and vinegar.

10. Cover the fish by lightly removing the excess marinade, dipping in the egg mixture, followed by the whey protein mixture, immediately putting it in hot oil and directly spraying the top. You want to cook the fish quickly after cooking to get the best sharpness. Cook on both sides until golden and place on a paper-covered plate for a few min

11. Serve immediately on a bed of potato chips with jicama, lots of lemons, mayonnaise and a pinch of vinegar.

Prep time: 20 min; **Servings:** 6

Macros: Cal 242 Fat 13 g Saturated fat 6 g Cholesterol 158 mg Sodium 427 mg Potassium 802 mg Carbs 1 g Sugar 1 g Protein 26 g

KETO CANNED TUNA PATTIES

Ingredients

- canned tuna

- 2 cups sweet potatoes (chopped)

- 1 red pepper (finely chopped)

- 1 yellow onion (chopped)

- 1 garlic clove (minced)

- ¼ cup chopped fresh chives

- ½ lime (juice)

- 1 egg

- ½ Tbsp salt (I used natural salt, so useless if you use fine cooking salt)

- ½ tsp ground black pepper

- 1 tsp bell pepper

Instructions

1. Cut the sweet potato into small cubes and cook in salted water for 10 min

2. While the sweet potato cooks, brown the chopped red pepper and onion in a little oil until the onion is tender.

3. Now mix everything in a bowl until it is well mixed.

4. Form the mixture into fish cookies. I used ¼ cup per cake, and this produced 12 cakes.

5. Heat the oil in a pan over medium heat. Once the pan is hot, carefully place the fish cakes in the pan and have them carefully monitored on each side. Let them sit for at least 3 min on each side.

Prep time: 10 min; **Servings:** 4

Macros: Cal 343 Carbs 18.4 g Protein 38.9 g Fat 12.2 g Saturated Fat 2.6 g Cholesterol 82 mg Sodium 977 mg Potassium 863 mg Fiber 3.5 g Sugar 6.7 g Calcium: 20 mg Iron: 3.6 mg

PAPILLOTE FISH

Ingredients

- ¾ lbs of white fish fillet such as bass, halibut or cod (boneless and skinless)

- 1-2 chopped chives bulbs

Sauce:

- 1 lemongrass stem

- 2 Tbsp olive oil

- 1.5 Tbsp red boat fish sauce

  - 1 large shallots, finely chopped

  - 1 ash or serrano red pepper, seedless and finely chopped (optional)

  - Black pepper to taste, optional

Crispy garlic cloves:

- large garlic cloves, thinly sliced

- avocado oil Tbsp

- Salt to taste

Instructions

1. Sauce: Preheat the oven to 400°F (200C). Remove the hard outer part of the lemongrass. Cut the green upper part and use only the white part with the lamp. Use a bottle or meat grinder to mash the lemongrass several times until it is flat, then chop it finely. Mix all the ingredients in "Salsa." Put aside.

2. In foil (parchment paper cover): Start with a sheet of parchment paper about 18 to 20 inches long. Fold it in half and open it again. Place the fish fillet in the center of the paper next to the folded edge. For the sauce over it.

3. Then fold the paper so that the 2 ends meet and surround the food. Start at both ends of the fold in the middle, make small diagonal folds on top of the filling, fold it on all sides to create an airtight semicircular packaging that looks like a crescent-shaped calzone. Close the foil tightly. You may need to turn and bend the tip to secure the envelope. Place the package on a large pan.

4. Cook at 400°F, on the upper rack, for 12-20 min (depending on the type and thickness of the fillets) until you obtain a flaky butter. Try a skewer; If it comes in quickly, the fish is ready. Let cool 3 to 4 min before using a pair of kitchen scissors to open the packaging (watch out for hot steam).

5. Crispy garlic: before the fish is finished cooking, heat a pan over medium heat until it is scorching. Add 2 Tbsp avocado oil and finely chopped garlic cloves. Use a wooden spoon to move gently and fry the slices in the pan until they are golden.

Servings: 2; **Prep time:** 10 min

Macros: Cal 443 Carbs 6 g Protein 31 g Fat 32 g saturated Fat 4 g Sugar 1 g

SUPER FISH VERACRUZ

Ingredients

- extra virgin olive oil Tbsp

- tilapia fillets (or other white fish)

- Really salty

- 1 yellow onion (thinly sliced)

- 1 Anaheim pepper (thinly sliced)

- 3 garlic cloves (thinly sliced)

- 2 bay leaves

- ½ tsp oregano (minced meat)

- cups oFresh tomatoes

- ¼ cup green olives

- 2 capers

- Lima (to serve)

Instructions

Pan method

1   Heat the oil in a large skillet until it is medium/high.

2   Salt and pepper on both sides of the fish press lightly with your fingertips.

3   Put the fish in the hot pan and cook for 3-4 minutes until lightly browned.

4   Gently turn the fish over and fry for 2 min on the other side.

5   Remove the fish and place it carefully on a plate.

6   Add the onion and chili to the pan and bake for 2-3 min, or until the onion begins to soften.

7   Add the garlic and fry for an additional 30 seconds.

8   Add bay leaves, oregano, crushed tomatoes, green olives, and capers.

9   Bring to a boil and cook about 5 min.

10 Return the fish to the pan and simmer for 3-4 min until the fish is thoroughly cooked. Remove bay leaves.

11 Serve with lemon slices.

Servings: 6; **Prep time:**10 min

Macros: Cal 176 Carbs 6 g Protein 25 g Fat 6.8 g saturated Fat 1.4 g

CREAMY AVOCADO CUCUMBER NOODLES WITH SMOKED SALMON

Ingredients

- 2 large cucumbers [hairspring]

- 2 large avocados

- 200 g smoked salmon

- 2 Tbsp lime juice [about ½ lime]

- 1 tsp dijon mustard

- 1 Tbsp olive oil

- 1 finely chopped garlic Tbsp

- to taste salt and pepper

- ½ optional onion [thinly sliced]

- ½ cup optional caper berries

- 4 Tbsp optional cream cheese

● 1 tsp black sesame seeds to garnish your choice

Instructions

7. Cut the cucumbers into noodles using a spiral. Then salt and set aside the noodles evenly.

8. Combine avocado, olive oil, mustard Dijon, lime juice, garlic, salt and pepper and blend until smooth.

9. Combine avocado sauce with the cucumber noodles until all the noodles are equally coated.

Servings: 4; **Prep time:** 15 min

Macros: Cal 370 Carbs 17.9 g Protein 13.6 g Fat 29.5 g Saturated Fat 7.4 g Fiber 8.5 g Sugar 3.8 g

FRIED FISH WITH MUSTARD

Ingredients

- ¼ cup chopped onion

- ½ tsp minced garlic (1 clove)

- 1 Tbsp butter or clarified oil

- 3 cups diced red potatoes

- ¼ cup chopped celery

- 2 cups Brussels sprouts (minced)

- ¼ tsp cayenne pepper or smoked paprika

- 2 cod fillets (4 oz-5 oz each)

- ¼ cup mustard vinaigrette (or 3 Tbsp honey or Dijon mustard with 1 Tbsp olive oil and 1 tsp red wine vinegar)

- Lemon juice and sliced lemons

- balsamic vinegar for watering

- salt and pepper to taste

- ⅓ cup parmesan or feta on top (skip for paleo option)

- Garnish with parsley and an extra lemon slice

Instructions

1. Wash and clean your vegetables and fish fillets.

2. Cut the potatoes into quarters and finely chop the sprouts or put them in a food processor to make crisps.

3. Then brown potatoes in 1 Tbsp oil or butter, ¼ cup onion, garlic, and a pinch of salt/pepper. Cook until the vegetables are slightly tender and the onions start to caramelize. About 10 min over medium heat.

4. Then cover the fillets with mustard vinaigrette and lemon juice and set aside.

5. Combine your vegetable and potato/onion mixture in a saucepan or frying pan. Make sure to put all the oil and garlic in the pan when you cook the potatoes.

6. Mix the vegetables with a little balsamic vinegar and herbs (paprika, salt, pepper, etc.). Put the fish fillets on top. Pour extra mustard and honey vinaigrette over the entire pan, which also covers the vegetables. Sprinkle with optional Parmesan or feta.

7. Bake for 14 to 17 min at 450°F. Check the vegetables after 14 min If it is tender, grill it at the last minute so that the sprouts are crisp!

8. Remove and garnish with red pepper flakes and parsley if desired. Salt/pepper to taste.

Servings: 4; **Prep time:** 15 min

Macros: Cal 237 Sugar 2.9 g Fat 9.4 g Saturated Fat 2 g Carbs 23.6 g Fiber 4.4 g Protein 17.4 g Cholesterol 32.9 mg

SMOKED SALMON WRAPS AND CUCUMBER

Ingredients

- slices of ham

- ½ cucumber, thinly sliced

- 100 g smoked salmon

- 1 Tbsp (15 ml) coconut cream

- Green salad to serve

Instructions

1 Spread the coconut cream on each slice of ham.

2 Place slices of smoked salmon on each slice of ham.

3 Place thin slices of cucumber on top.

4 Roll up the wrap and place it on the green salad to serve.

Prep time: 5 min; **Serving Size:** 2 wraps

Macros: Cal 210 Sugar 0 g Fat 10 g Carbs 0 g Fiber 0 g Protein 29 g

MINI FISH COOKIES

Ingredients

- 1 lb Fresh white fish made into a paste

- 2 cups almond flour

- 4 eggs, beaten

- 1 Tbsp lemon juice or white wine vinegar

- 1 tsp of baking powder

- 2 spoonfuls of chives or spring onions, finely chopped

- 1 spoonful of garlic powder

- 1 spoonful of butter or coconut oil

- To taste salt and pepper

Instructions

6. Preheat the oven to 190 ° C.

7. In a large bowl, add all the ingredients.

8. Place the muffin tins on a muffin tray and add the mixture to each pan.

9. Bake till the mini fish patties are firm and golden on top for 25 min.

Prep time: 10 min;

Macros: Cal 120 Sugar 0 g Fat 8 g Carbs 2 g Fiber 1 g Protein 11 g

TRADITIONAL CHINESE STEAMED WHOLE GINGER FISH

Ingredients

- 1 whole fish, clean

- 1 tsp salt

- ½ cup spring onions, cut into thin strips (divide into 2 parts)

- 2 Tbsp ginger, cut into small pieces (divided into 2 parts)

- ½ cup tamari soy sauce

- 1 Tbsp avocado oil

- 2 red peppers, sliced

- 20 Sichuan peppercorns

- 1 Tbsp sesame oil

Instructions

1. Clean the fish (remove the scales and the interior) (or ask your fishmonger to clean it for you). You can cut your head

off if you want and use it to make fish soup. Cut slits on both sides of the fish and rub it with salt.

2. Place the fish on a plate and for ¼ cup tamari soy sauce (or coconut amino acids) over the fish with half the spring onion and ginger. Place water in your evaporator: place the plate on the evaporator when the water begins to boil.

3. Steam for 12 min

4. For the avocado oil into a saucepan over high heat. Add the Sichuan peppercorns, peppers, and the rest of the ginger and chives.

5. Prepare the new sauce with the rest of tamari soy sauce (¼ cup) and sesame oil.

6. Remove the steamed fish (discard the sauce in which the fish was cooked). For the new sauce over fish, cover with the roasted chili, ginger, and chives and serve.

Prep time:15 min; **Servings:** 2

Macros: Cal 110 Fat 4 g Carbs 2 g Protein 14 g

SARDINES WITH OLIVES

Ingredients

- 1 Tbsp (15 ml) olive oil

- 5 black olives in slices.

- 1 Tbsp (1 g) Flakes of parsley.

- 1 Tbsp (6 g) Flakes of garlic.

- 1 can of sardines (100 g each).

Instructions

7. Place the olive oil and garlic in the pan and fry for 5 min.

8. Add the can of sardines and olives and cook for 8 min.

9. Finally, add parsley and serve.

Prep time: 5 min; **Servings:** 2

Macros: Cal 416 Sugar 2g Fat 33g Carbs 7g Fiber 2g Protein 21g Net Carbs 5 g

SMOKED TUNA PICKLES

Ingredients

6. 2 6-oz cans (or bags) of bluefin tuna

7. 1 6-oz can (or bag) smoked tuna

8. ⅓ cup unsweetened mayonnaise

9. 1 Tbsp dried onion flakes (or ½ tsp onion powder)

10. ¼ tsp garlic powder

11. ¼ tsp ground black pepper

12. 6 large whole pickles

Instructions

1. Combine all ingredients except pickles in a medium bowl and mix well.

2. Cut the pickles in half and gently remove the seeds from the middle.

3. Place about 3 Tbsp (more or less) of tuna salad in each half of the pickle.

4. Let cool and serve.

Prep time: 5 min;

Macros: Cal 118 Fat 7 g Carbs 1.5 g net Protein 11 g

GARLIC LIME MAHI-MAHI

Ingredients

3. ¼ C avocado oil

4. Last of a lime

5. Lime juice

6. garlic cloves, finely chopped

7. A pinch oFine grain sea salt

8. A pinch of ground black pepper

9. Mahi-Mahi steaks (1 - 1 ¼ lb)

Instructions

1. Mix everything except the fillets in a small bowl to make the marinade.

2. Pour over the steaks in a large shallow dish or in a large airtight bag. Leave to marinate for 30 minutes.

3. Pour the marinade into a pan for cooking (with a lid). Heat the liquid over medium heat. Carefully place the fillets in the pan, cover, and cook for 4 min

4. Remove from heat and let stand for 5 min

Prep time: 10 min; **Servings:** 2-4

Macros: Cal 95 Carbs 0 g Fat 1 g Protein 10 g

CREAMY LEEK AND SALMON SOUP

Ingredients

- 2 Tbsp avocado oil

- 4 leeks, washed, cut into half moons

- 3 garlic cloves, finely chopped

- 6 cups seafood or chicken broth

- 2 tsp dried thyme leaves

- 1 lb salmon, cut into small pieces

- 1 3/4 cups coconut milk

- Salt and pepper to taste

Instructions

1. Heat the avocado oil in a large saucepan or in the Dutch oven over medium heat.

2. Add the chopped leek and garlic and cook until tender.

3. For the broth and add the thyme. Cook over low heat for about 15 min and season with salt and pepper.

4. Put the salmon and coconut milk in the pan. Simmer again and simmer until the fish is opaque and soft.

Servings: 4; **Prep time:**10 min

Macros: 240 Fat 11 g saturated 6 g Carbs 23 g Sugar 2 g Fiber 3 g Protein 14 g salt 1.58 g

MOQUECA - BRAZILIAN FISH STEW

Ingredients

Soup:

- ½ to 2 lbs of solid white fish fillets such as halibut, swordfish or cod, rinsed in cold water

- boneless, cut into large portions

- 3 garlic cloves, finely chopped

- 4 Tbsp lime or lemon juice

- Salt

- Freshly ground black pepper

- Extra virgin olive oil

- 1 cup chopped sweet onion or 1 medium yellow onion, chopped or sliced

- ¼ cup chopped green onion leaves

- ½ yellow bell pepper and ½ red bell pepper, seedless, inflamed, finely chopped (or sliced)

- 2 cups chopped tomatoes (or sliced)

- 1 Tbsp sweet pepper

- 1 pinch of red pepper flakes

- 1 large bunch of coriander, to garnish

- 1 can (14 oz) coconut milk

Instructions

7. Cover the fish with garlic and lime juice: put the pieces oFish in a bowl, add the chopped garlic and lime juice so that the pieces are well covered. Generously sprinkle with salt and pepper.

8. Chill while you prepare the rest of the soup.

9. Cook the onion, pepper, tomatoes, green onions: put about 2 Tbsp olive oil in a large covered pan over medium heat.

10. Add chopped onion and jumped for a few min until it is tender. Add the bell pepper, bell pepper, and red pepper flakes. Sprinkle generously with salt and pepper. (At least a tsp salt). Cook for a few more minutes until the pepper begins to soften.

11. Add the chopped tomatoes and onion vegetables. Bring to a boil and cook uncovered for 5 min Add chopped cilantro.

12. Place the vegetables with fish, add the coconut milk: use a large spoon to remove about half of the vegetables (you replace them). Spread the remaining vegetables at the bottom of the pan to create a bed for the fish.

13. Mix the pieces of fish with vegetables. Season with salt and pepper. Then add the vegetables

14. Pour the coconut milk over the fish and vegetables.

15. Simmer, cook, adjust the spices: bring the soup to a boil, reduce the heat, cover and simmer for 15 min. Taste and regulate the herbs.

16. You may need to add more salt, lime or lemon juice, pepper, pepper, or chili flakes to get the flavor you want.

17. Garnish with cilantro.

Prep time: 10 min; **Servings:** 5

Macros: 291 Fat 8.1 g Saturated 5.4 g Sugar 8.5 g

SMOKED SALMON SALAD WITH PINK PEPPER

Ingredients

- 1 handful arugula lettuce leaves

- 1 tsp lightly ground pink peppercorns

- 4 olives

- 50 g of smoked salmon

- 1 lemon slice

Instructions

1. Place the arugula lettuce leaves and olives in a shallow bowl or dish.

2. Place the smoked salmon on the salad.

3. Sprinkle lightly ground rose seeds on smoked salmon.

4. Garnish with a lemon slice and serve immediately.

Prep time:5 min; **Servings:** 1

Macros: Cal 117 Carbs 1 g Fat 6 g Protein 16 g

MOJO GARLIC FISH FILLET

Ingredients

- 1½ tilapia or other fish fillets

- 1 lime

- Salt and pepper to taste

- ¼ cup vegetable oil (or a mixture of half olive oil and half

- vegetable oil)

- 6 garlic cloves, thinly sliced

- 3 finely chopped parsley Tbsp

- 2 Tbsp optional flour, see note

Instructions

1. Season the fish with salt, pepper, and lemon juice. Reserve while you prepare the rest of the ingredients.

2. Heat the oil over low heat in a large skillet. Cook the golden garlic slices as soon as they are hot. Be sure to remove them

quickly as soon as they are light brown; If you leave them longer, they will taste bitter. This step takes a few seconds, so be careful.

3. If you are using flour, sprinkle the flour fillets very lightly. Put the heat on medium-high in the pan where you cooked garlic. Add the fish and fry on both sides. The cooking time depends on the thickness of the fish. It takes about 2-3 min

4. about ⅓ inch thick per side for these steaks, and about 5-7 min for thicker steaks. Do not turn the fish until all sides are brown and cooked.

5. Remove it from the pan and place it on a cooling rack with a paper towel underneath to absorb excess fat. Garnish with chopped parsley and golden garlic slices to serve.

Prep time: 10 min; **Serving Size:** 6 oz

Macros: Cal 307 Carbs 6g Protein 35g Fat 16g Saturated Fat 12g

SELTZER FISH

Ingredients

4. 1 lb cod or salmon, cut into pieces oFish sticks

5. 3/4 tsp dried dill, optional for seasoning fish

6. ¼ cup + 2 Tbsp cassava flour, divided

7. ¼ cup coconut flour

8. 2 Tb + 2 Tb tapioca starch, divided

9. ½ tsp Himalayan salt

10. 1 cup flavored mineral water, such as La Croix or Perrier

11. 3 to 4 cups of oil for high frying heat, such as refined avocado oil or refined olive oil

Instructions

1. Season the fish pieces with dill if desired and keep them in the fridge while you prepare the other ingredients. This helps the fish not to overcook while it is being cooked later.

2. Heat the oil in a medium stainless steel pot with high sides to around 375 F. You want oil at least 4 "deep so that the dough does not stick to the bottom of the pan.

3. Make a plate lined with paper towels and place it on your kitchen counter near the jar.

4. Combine ¼ cup cassava flour, all of the coconut flour, 2 Tbsp tapioca starch, and salt in a medium bowl. It will be for your drummer.

5. Combine the remaining 2 Tbsp cassava flour and 2 Tbsp tapioca starch in a small bowl. It is to sprinkle the fish before it hits it. It helps the dough to adhere better to the fish.

6. Add a little seltzer to the flour in a medium bowl with a fork. Work carefully through the pieces until you have a soft dough that barely slides from the back of a spoon. You may not need all the seltzer or something extra, depending on the flower brands you use.

7. Roll about 4 or 5 pieces oFish at a time in the smallest dish with sprinkled flour.

8. Now use a fork or spoon to roll the pieces into the dough.

9. Carefully place each piece oFish with long tongs in the hot oil. Do not overfill the pot. Otherwise, you will get soaked fish that will not break.

10. Bake for about 4 to 5 min, turning them occasionally with the tongs to prevent them from sticking evenly and turning brown.

11. Place the crispy fish on a plate with paper towels.

12. Repeat the process of dusting, dough, and fry 4 to 5 pieces at a time.

13. If you still have dough and flour to sprinkle, mix them and use a spoon to form in the hot oil little by little, and voila, now you also have crispy and delicious donuts!

Prep time: 10 min; **Servings:** 2

Macros: Cal 257 Carbs 4g Protein 25g Fat 6g Saturated Fat 5g

GRILLED WHITE FISH WITH ZUCCHINI AND KALE PESTO

Ingredients

- Kale pesto

- 3 g of kale

- 3 Tbsp lime juice or juice

- 2 g of nuts

- 1 of the best clothes

- ½ tsp

- ¼ tsp ground blüker black

- Olive oil C cup

- Fish and zucchini

- 2 zuchini

- 1 Tbsp lemon juice

- ½ tsp salt

- 2 Tbsp oil

- 1½ lbs oFish

- ¼ tsp black pepper

Instructions

6. Put the kale, walnuts, lime, and garlic in a blender or food processor and puree until smooth. Season with salt and pepper.

7. Rinse the zuchín and cut it fine with a knife, a cutting machine, or a pipe. Place the slices in a cave. Season with salt and pepper to taste and dry with olives and olive oil. Add rest on both sides and sit for a few min Clean off excess liquid and rinse with oil.

8. Grill or a few min on each side. Add pepper and serve with zucchini and pesto.

Prep time: 10 min; **Servings:** 4

Macros: Carbs (7 g) Fiber 3 g Fat (67 g) Protein (38 g) Cal 778

GRILLED SALMON WITH GINGER SAUCE

Ingredients:

- 1 tablespoon toasted sesame oil

- 1 tablespoon fresh cilantro, chopped

- 1 tablespoon lime juice

- 1 teaspoon fish sauce

- 1 clove garlic, mashed

- 1 teaspoon fresh ginger, grated

- 1 teaspoon jalapeño pepper, minced

- 4 salmon fillets

- 1 tablespoon olive oil

- Salt and pepper to taste

Instructions

1. In a bowl, mix the sesame oil, cilantro, lime juice, fish sauce, garlic, ginger and jalapeño pepper.

2. Preheat your grill.

3. Brush oil on salmon.

4. Season both sides with salt and pepper.

5. Grill salmon for 6 to 8 minutes, turning once or twice.

6. Take 1 tablespoon from the oil mixture.

7. Brush this on the salmon while grilling.

8. Serve grilled salmon with the remaining sauce.

Preparation Time: 15 minutes **Servings:** 4

Cooking Time: 8 minutes

Nutrition: Calories 204 Total Fat 11 g Saturated Fat 2 g Cholesterol 53 mg Sodium 320 mg Total Carbohydrate 2 g Dietary Fiber 0 g Total Sugars 2 g Protein 23 g Potassium 437 mg

ALMOND CRUSTED BAKED CHILI MAHI MAHI

Ingredients:

- 4 mahi mahi fillets

- 1 lime

- 2 teaspoons olive oil

- Salt and pepper to taste

- ½ cup almonds

- ¼ teaspoon paprika

- ¼ teaspoon onion powder

- ¾ teaspoon chili powder

- ½ cup red bell pepper, chopped

- ¼ cup onion, chopped

- ¼ cup fresh cilantro, chopped

Instructions

1. Preheat your oven to 325 degrees F.

2. Line your baking pan with parchment paper.

3. Squeeze juice from the lime.

4. Grate zest from the peel.

5. Put juice and zest in a bowl.

6. Add the oil, salt and pepper.

7. In another bowl, add the almonds, paprika, onion powder and chili powder.

8. Put the almond mixture in a food processor.

9. Pulse until powdery.

10. Dip each fillet in the oil mixture.

11. Dredge with the almond and chili mixture.

12. Arrange on a single layer in the oven.

13. Bake for 12 to 15 minutes or until fully cooked.

14. Serve with red bell pepper, onion and cilantro.

Preparation Time: 20 minutes **Servings:** 4

Cooking Time: 15 minutes

Nutrition: Calories 322 Total Fat 12 g Saturated Fat 2 g Cholesterol 83 mg Sodium 328 mg Total Carbohydrate 28 g Dietary Fiber 4 g Total Sugars 10 g Protein 28 g Potassium 829 mg

SWORDFISH WITH TOMATO SALSA

Ingredients:

- 1 cup tomato, chopped

- ¼ cup tomatillo, chopped

- 2 tablespoons fresh cilantro, chopped

- ¼ cup avocado, chopped

- 1 clove garlic, minced

- 1 jalapeño pepper, chopped

- 1 tablespoon lime juice

- Salt and pepper to taste

- 4 swordfish steaks

- 1 clove garlic, sliced in half

- 2 tablespoons lemon juice

- ½ teaspoon ground cumin

Instructions

1. Preheat your grill.

2. In a bowl, mix the tomato, tomatillo, cilantro, avocado, garlic, jalapeño, lime juice, salt and pepper.

3. Cover the bowl with foil and put in the refrigerator.

4. Rub each swordfish steak with sliced garlic.

5. Drizzle lemon juice on both sides.

6. Season with salt, pepper and cumin.

7. Grill for 12 minutes or until the fish is fully cooked.

8. Serve with salsa.

Preparation Time: 20 minutes **Servings:** 4

Cooking Time: 12 minutes

Nutrition: Calories 190 Total Fat 8 g Saturated Fat 2 g Cholesterol 43 mg Sodium 254 mg Total Carbohydrate 6 g Dietary Fiber 3 g Total Sugars 1 g Protein 24 g Potassium 453 mg

SALMON & ASPARAGUS

Ingredients:

- 2 salmon fillets

- 8 spears asparagus, trimmed

- 2 tablespoons balsamic vinegar

- 1 teaspoon olive oil

- 1 teaspoon dried dill

- Salt and pepper to taste

Instructions

1. Preheat your oven to 325 degrees F.

2. Dry salmon with paper towels.

3. Arrange the asparagus around the salmon fillets on a baking pan.

4. In a bowl, mix the rest of the ingredients.

5. Pour mixture over the salmon and vegetables.

6. Bake in the oven for 10 minutes or until the fish is fully cooked.

Preparation Time: 15 minutes **Servings:** 2

Cooking Time: 10 minutes

Nutrition: Calories 328 Total Fat 15 g Saturated Fat 3 g Cholesterol 67 mg Sodium 365 mg Total Carbohydrate 6 g Dietary Fiber 4 g Total Sugars 5 g Protein 28 g Potassium 258 mg

HALIBUT WITH SPICY APRICOT SAUCE

Ingredients:

- 4 fresh apricots, pitted

- 1/3 cup apricot preserves

- ½ cup apricot nectar

- ½ teaspoon dried oregano

- 3 tablespoons scallion, sliced

- 1 teaspoon hot pepper sauce

- Salt to taste

- 4 halibut steaks

- 1 tablespoon olive oil

Instructions

3. Put the apricots, preserves, nectar, oregano, scallion, hot pepper sauce and salt in a saucepan.

4. Bring to a boil and then simmer for 8 minutes.

5. Set aside.

6. Brush the halibut steaks with olive oil.

7. Grill for 7 to 9 minutes or until fish is flaky.

8. Brush one tablespoon of the sauce on both sides of the fish.

9. Serve with the reserved sauce.

Preparation Time: 15 minutes **Servings:** 4

Cooking Time: 17 minutes

Nutrition: Calories 304 Total Fat 8 g Saturated Fat 1 g Cholesterol 73 mg Sodium 260 mg Total Carbohydrate 27 g Dietary Fiber 2 g Total Sugars 16 g Protein 29 g Potassium 637 mg

POPCORN SHRIMP

Ingredients:

- Cooking spray

- ½ cup all-purpose flour

- 2 eggs, beaten

- 2 tablespoons water

- 1 ½ cups panko breadcrumbs

- 1 tablespoon garlic powder

- 1 tablespoon ground cumin

- 1 lb. shrimp, peeled and deveined

- ½ cup ketchup

- 2 tablespoons fresh cilantro, chopped

- 2 tablespoons lime juice

- Salt to taste

Instructions

1. Coat the air fryer basket with cooking spray

2. Put the flour in a dish.

3. In the second dish, beat the eggs and water.

4. In the third dish, mix the breadcrumbs, garlic powder and cumin.

5. Dip each shrimp in each of the three dishes, first in the dish with flour, then the egg and then breadcrumb mixture.

6. Place the shrimp in the air fryer basket.

7. Cook at 360 degrees F for 8 minutes, flipping once halfway through.

8. Combine the rest of the ingredients as dipping sauce for the shrimp.

Preparation Time: 15 minutes **Servings:** 4

Cooking Time: 8 minutes

Nutrition: Calories 297 Total Fat 4 g Saturated Fat 1 g Cholesterol 276 mg Sodium 291 mg Total Carbohydrate 35 g Dietary Fiber 1 g Total Sugars 9 g Protein 29 g Potassium 390 mg

SHRIMP LEMON KEBAB

Ingredients:

- 1 ½ lb. shrimp, peeled and deveined but with tails intact

- 1/3 cup olive oil

- ¼ cup lemon juice

- 2 teaspoons lemon zest

- 1 tablespoon fresh parsley, chopped

- 8 cherry tomatoes, quartered

- 2 scallions, sliced

Instructions

1. Mix the olive oil, lemon juice, lemon zest and parsley in a bowl.

2. Marinate the shrimp in this mixture for 15 minutes.

3. Thread each shrimp into the skewers.

4. Grill for 4 to 5 minutes, turning once halfway through.

5. Serve with tomatoes and scallions.

Preparation Time: 10 minutes **Servings:** 4

Cooking Time: 5 minutes

Nutrition: Calories 271 Total Fat 12 g Saturated Fat 2 g Cholesterol 259 mg Sodium 255 mg Total Carbohydrate 4 g Dietary Fiber 1 g Total Sugars 1 g Protein 25 g Potassium 429 mg

Grilled Herbed Salmon with Raspberry Sauce & Cucumber Dill Dip

Ingredients:

- 3 salmon fillets

- 1 tablespoon olive oil

- Salt and pepper to taste

- 1 teaspoon fresh sage, chopped

- 1 tablespoon fresh parsley, chopped

- 2 tablespoons apple juice

- 1 cup raspberries

- 1 teaspoon Worcestershire sauce

- 1 cup cucumber, chopped

- 2 tablespoons light mayonnaise

- ½ teaspoon dried dill

Instructions

1. Coat the salmon fillets with oil.

2. Season with salt, pepper, sage and parsley.

3. Cover the salmon with foil.

4. Grill for 20 minutes or until fish is flaky.

5. While waiting, mix the apple juice, raspberries and Worcestershire sauce.

6. Pour the mixture into a saucepan over medium heat.

7. Bring to a boil and then simmer for 8 minutes.

8. In another bowl, mix the rest of the ingredients.

9. Serve salmon with raspberry sauce and cucumber dip.

Preparation Time: 15 minutes **Servings:** 4

Cooking Time: 30 minutes

Nutrition: Calories 256 Total Fat 15 g Saturated Fat 3 g Cholesterol 68 mg Sodium 176 mg Total Carbohydrate 6 g Dietary Fiber 1 g Total Sugars 5 g Protein 23 g Potassium 359 mg

TARRAGON SCALLOPS

Ingredients:

- 1 cup water

- 1 lb. asparagus spears, trimmed

- 2 lemons

- 1 ¼ lb. scallops

- Salt and pepper to taste

- 1 tablespoon olive oil

- 1 tablespoon fresh tarragon, chopped

Instructions

1. Pour water into a pot.

2. Bring to a boil.

3. Add asparagus spears.

4. Cover and cook for 5 minutes.

5. Drain and transfer to a plate.

6. Slice one lemon into wedges.

7. Squeeze juice and shred zest from the remaining lemon.

8. Season the scallops with salt and pepper.

9. Put a pan over medium heat.

10. Add oil to the pan.

11. Cook the scallops until golden brown.

12. Transfer to the same plate, putting scallops beside the asparagus.

13. Add lemon zest, juice and tarragon to the pan.

14. Cook for 1 minute.

15. Drizzle tarragon sauce over the scallops and asparagus.

Preparation Time: 10 minutes **Servings:** 4

Cooking Time: 15 minutes

Nutrition: Calories 253 Total Fat 12 g Saturated Fat 2 g Cholesterol 47 mg Sodium 436 mg Total Carbohydrate 14 g Dietary Fiber 5 g Total Sugars 3 g Protein 27 g Potassium 773 mg

GARLIC SHRIMP & SPINACH

Ingredients:

- 3 tablespoons olive oil, divided

- 6 clove garlic, sliced and divided

- 1 lb. spinach

- Salt to taste

- 1 tablespoons lemon juice

- 1 lb. shrimp, peeled and deveined

- ¼ teaspoon red pepper, crushed

- 1 tablespoon parsley, chopped

- 1 teaspoon lemon zest

Instructions

1. Pour 1 tablespoon olive oil in a pot over medium heat.

2. Cook the garlic for 1 minute.

3. Add the spinach and season with salt.

4. Cook for 3 minutes.

5. Stir in lemon juice.

6. Transfer to a bowl.

7. Pour the remaining oil.

8. Add the shrimp.

9. Season with salt and add red pepper.

10. Cook for 5 minutes.

11. Sprinkle parsley and lemon zest over the shrimp before serving.

Preparation Time: 10 minutes **Servings:** 4

Cooking Time: 10 minutes

Nutrition: Calories 226 Total Fat 12 g Saturated Fat 2 g Cholesterol 183 mg Sodium 444 mg Total Carbohydrate 6 g Dietary Fiber 3 g Total Sugars 1 g Protein 26 g Potassium 963 m

CONCLUSION

We've reached the end of this journey to the bottom of the sea, through the waves and into your board. Have you practiced cooking these delicacies to the best of your ability? Have you shared these dishes with family and friends?

Seafood always requires a little attention and practice, but if you practice cooking you will become a perfect keto chef.

I always recommend that you consult a doctor or nutritionist before committing to a diet and always stay healthy.

I embrace you and look forward to the next flavor journey.

CPSIA information can be obtained
at www.ICGtesting.com
Printed in the USA
LVHW011634020421
683321LV00004B/762

9 781678 052058